Pharmacy Law

By Babir Malik

Text copyright © 2020 Babir Malik
All Rights Reserved

About the author

Babir studied pharmacy at the University of Bradford and graduated in 2007 (after previously studying Biomedical Sciences at the same university). He joined Weldricks Pharmacy as a summer student in 2005, undertook his pre-reg with them and has stayed with them ever since.

Babir is now the Weldricks Pre-reg and Pharmacy Student Lead and Weldricks Teacher Practitioner, at the University of Bradford. He is also the Green Light Campus Northern Pre-Reg Lead, PCPA National Pre-reg Lead, Charity Ambassador for Pharmacist Support, Associate Fellow at HEA, as well as a tutor on the Royal Pharmaceutical Society Pre-Registration Conferences.

Babir currently practices as a relief pharmacist for Weldricks. In June 2016, the pharmacy that he co-managed at the time was awarded the Chemist and Druggist Medicines Optimisation Award for their innovative Local Pharmaceutical Service Intervention Service. He is a Chemist and Druggist Clinical Advisory Board Member.

As a Teacher Practitioner, his role includes being the final year Calculations Lead. Furthermore, Babir undertook a 10-week secondment as a Clinical Commissioning Group Pharmacist in North Lincolnshire early in 2016. He is also an OnTrack question writer and reviewer and is on the Medicines, Ethics and Practice Advisory Group. He completed his Clinical Diploma in Community Pharmacy at the University of Keele.

He can be found quite often on Twitter @Babir1981

Preface

While Pharmacy Law is not always the most exciting of topics it is a vital part of pharmacy, especially community pharmacy.

This book should be used after you have read the MEP or your lecture notes and before attempting law multiple choice questions. It is also a fun way of refreshing your knowledge as pharmacist or pharmacy technician and could be used as tool to aid revision for the registration assessment.

This book is not endorsed by the Royal Pharmaceutical Society or General Pharmaceutical Council.

This book was written using MEP 43 and was correct at the time of publication. There are no worked answers and if you are unsure after seeing the correct answer then please refer to the latest MEP.

If you have any comments, questions or suggestions for topics then I can be contacted on
pharmacylawquizzes@gmail.com

Babir Malik

Foreword

I have known Babir since his days as his alter-ego, the undercover writer Mr Dispenser. His love for pharmacy was evident even as he poked gentle fun at the idiosyncrasies found within the profession.

A few years on, Babir has taken to channelling this passion to support the next generation of pharmacists. His is a name well-known to students and trainees either through his numerous teaching roles, his social media presence, or via the multitude of online groups he moderates that support learners at various stages of their pharmacy careers.

And so we come to the latest addition to his growing collection of pharmacy-related books: Pharmacy Law Quizzes. The importance of law to our work should not be underestimated; it underpins our activity as pharmacists and provides an important part of the framework around which we assess our scope of practice.

I hope this book provides a helpful reference point for your current stage of understanding and facilitates the identification of any knowledge gaps that can be targeted for further study.

Atif Shamim

Associate Head of Pharmacy, Health Education England London, Kent Surrey and Sussex

National Professional Lead, Pre-registration Pharmacist Recruitment Scheme

Acknowledgements

I would like to thank Joanna Domzal-Jamroz, Kat Thorne and Emma Fielding for their kind assistance.

Glossary

CD: Controlled drugs
EEA: European Economic Area
EHC: Emergency Hormonal Contraception
GMC: General Medical Council
GSL: General Sales List
MEP: Medicines, Ethics and Practice
MHRA: Medicines and Healthcare products Regulatory Agency
NFA-VPS: Non-Food Animal – Veterinarian, Pharmacist, Suitably Qualified Person
OTC: Over the Counter
P: Pharmacy medicine
PGD: Patient Group Direction.
POM: Prescription-only Medicine
POM-V: Prescription-only Medicine – Veterinarian
POM-VPS: Prescription-only Medicine – Veterinarian, Pharmacist, Suitably Qualified Person
PPP: Pregnancy Prevention Programme
PSD: Patient Specific Direction
RP: Responsible Pharmacist
RPS: Royal Pharmaceutical Society

1. GSL medicines can only be sold from a pharmacy: True or False?

2. P medicines can be available for self-selection: True or False?

3. A physiotherapist independent prescriber can prescribe schedule 2 CDs: True or False?

4. It is unlawful to sell a product that contains more than 600 mg of pseudoephedrine: True or False?

5. Advanced supply of EHC is allowed: True or False?

6. Ulipristal acetate is only licensed for emergency contraception within 72 hours of unprotected sexual intercourse: True or False?

7. The legal limit of paracetamol effervescent tablets that can be sold is 100: True or False?

8. The maximum pack size for OTC dihydrocodeine is 16: True or False?

9. The date of birth is a legal requirement on a prescription for a POM: True or False?

10. The name of the prescriber is a legal requirement on a prescription: True or False?

11. All prescriptions are valid for up to 6 months from the appropriate date: True or False?

12. It is not a legal requirement for all prescriptions to be written in English: True or False?

13. Private prescriptions for Schedule 4 and 5 CDs cannot be repeated: True or False?

14. The first dispensing of a private prescription must be made within 6 months of the appropriate date, following which there is no legal time limit for the remaining repeats: True or False?

15. NHS prescriptions can be repeated: True or False?

16. Owings for co-codamol 30/500 tablets are valid for 28 days from the appropriate date: True or False?

17. The name of the drug is a legal requirement for a POM: True or False?

18. Private prescriptions for a POM must be retained for 2 years after dispensing: True or False?

19. Private prescriptions for oral contraceptives are exempt from record keeping: True or False?

20. The dose is a legal requirement when making a private prescription record in the POM register: True or False?

21. Schedule 2, 3, 4 and 5 CD owings are valid for 28 days after the appropriate date: True or False?

22. Faxed prescriptions are legal: True or False?

23. Dentists are only legally allowed to prescribe medicines on the Dental Practitioners Formulary: True or False?

24. A patient's date of birth is a legal requirement on an EEA prescription: True or False?

25. The prescriber's email address is a legal requirement on an EEA prescription: True or False?

26. The name of the drug is a legal requirement on an EEA prescription: True or False?

27. EEA prescriptions are subject to prescription charges: True or False?

28. Schedule 1, 2 and 3 CDs are not allowed on an EEA prescription: True or False?

29. Emergency supply at the request of an EEA prescriber is allowed: True or False?

30. Emergency supply at the request of an EEA patient for phenobarbital for epilepsy is allowed: True or False?

31. It is a legal requirement for the name of the doctor to appear on a dispensing label: True or False?

32. A patient specific direction is a written direction that allows the supply and/or administration of a specified medicine or medicines, by named authorised health professionals, to a well-defined group of patients requiring treatment for a specific condition: True or False?

33. In an emergency, a pharmacist working in a registered pharmacy can supply POMs to a animal without a prescription: True or False?

34. A podiatrist independent prescriber can request an emergency supply: True or False?

35. In an emergency supply at the request of a prescriber, the prescriber must furnish a prescription within 48 hours: True or False?

36. When making a POM register entry for an emergency supply at a request of a prescriber, two dates should be entered: True or False?

37. Legislation prevents a pharmacist from making an emergency supply when the doctor's surgery is open: True or False?

38. An emergency supply of phenobarbital in the UK can only be supplied for a maximum of 5 days: True or False?

39. When making a POM register entry for emergency supply at the request of a prescriber, the dose is a legal requirement: True or False?

40. All optometrists and podiatrists can authorise supplies of POMs by writing prescriptions: True or False?

41. Any schoolteacher can sign a signed order to obtain salbutamol inhalers: True or False?

42. The names of the students needing the salbutamol inhalers should be on the signed order: True or False?

43. Appropriately headed paper must be used on a signed order for adrenaline auto-injectors for a school: True or False?

44. Any pharmacist can supply nasal naloxone to a substance misuser without a prescription, PSD or PGD: True or False?

45. All female patients wanting isotretinoin prescriptions must comply with the Pregnancy Prevention Programme [PPP]: True or False?

46. Under the PPP, prescriptions for acitretin are valid for 7 days: True or False?

47. All prescriptions for isotretinoin should only be prescribed for 30 days: True or False?

48. Those planning pregnancies and taking valproate must schedule an appointment with their prescriber and stop taking valproate immediately: True or False?

49. Lantus™ is an example of an original biologic medicine: True or False?

50. A Pharmacist Independent Prescriber can prescribe unlicensed medicines subject to accepted good clinical practice: True or False?

51. An optometrist independent prescriber can authorise an emergency supply for items that they can prescribe: True or False?

52. A Vet can authorise an emergency supply for items that they can prescribe: True or False?

53. Pharmacies can supply appropriate health professionals with a small number of POMs via wholesale dealing as long as only a small profit is made: True or False?

54. An independent nurse prescriber can be supplied with a small amount of medicines via wholesale dealing: True or False?

55. POM-VPS are prescription-only medicines that can only be prescribed by a Vet and supplied by a Vet or pharmacist with a written prescription: True or False?

56. A written prescription is needed to supply a NFA-VPS medicine: True or False?

57. Vet prescriptions for Schedule 2, 3 and 4 drugs are valid for 28 days: True or False?

58. The Veterinary Medicines Directorate advise that "as directed" is a legally acceptable dosage instruction on a vet prescription: True or False?

59. Standardised forms are required for Vet schedule 2 and 3 CD prescriptions: True or False?

60. Vet CD prescriptions should be sent to the relevant NHS agency: True or False?

61. For all CDs, it is considered good practice for only 28 days' worth of treatment to be prescribed on a vet prescription: True or False?

62. All vet prescriptions must include the Royal College of Veterinary Surgeons Registration number of the Vet: True or False?

63. The cascade exemption within the Veterinary Medicines Regulations allows the supply of medicines that are not licensed for animals: True or False?

64. It is lawful to sell human medicines for use in animals: True or False?

65. The expiry date of a medicine supplied under the cascade must always be on the dispensing label: True or False?

66. An entry must be made in the POM register for all POM-V and POM-VPS: True or False?

67. Register entries for POM-V and POM-VPS can be kept electronically: True or False?

68. Records and documents for POM-V and POM-VPS must be kept for two years: True or False?

69. Animal adverse reactions and human adverse reactions to vet medicines should be reported to the MHRA: True or False?

70. The Health Act 2006 introduced the concept of an accountable officer: True or False?

71. There are two classes of Schedule 5 drugs: True or False?

72. Sativex is a Schedule 4 Part II drug: True or False?

73. Prescriptions for zopiclone are only valid for 28 days: True or False?

74. The address of prescriber for a schedule 4 CD must be in the UK: True or False?

75. NICE advise that organisations should consider retaining all CD invoices for six years for the purposes of HM Revenue and Customs: True or False?

76. Pharmacists can, under one specific exemption, take possession of a schedule 1 CD: True or False?

77. The name of supplier is a legal requirement for a CD requisition: True or False?

78. The total quantity of a drug in words and figures is a legal requirement for a CD requisition: True or False?

79. In an emergency, a doctor or dentist can be supplied with a Schedule 2 or 3 CD on the undertaking that a requisition will be supplied within the next 24 hours: True or False?

80. When a requisition for a schedule 1, 2 or 3 CD is received, it is a legal requirement to mark the requisition indelibly with the supplier's name and address: True or False?

81. The person requesting the CD must send the original requisition to the relevant NHS agency: True or False?

82. A registered midwife may use a midwife supply order to obtain diamorphine, morphine and oxycodone: True or False?

83. The name of prescriber is a legal requirement on a prescription for a schedule 2 or 3 CD: True or False?

84. The dose on a schedule 2 or 3 CD prescription does not need to be in words and figures: True or False?

85. The name of drug is not a legal requirement on a schedule 2 or 3 CD prescription: True or False?

86. It is a legal requirement for schedule 2, 3 or 4 CD prescriptions to not exceed a 30-day supply: True or False?

87. When a schedule 2 or 3 CD is supplied, it is a requirement to mark the prescription with the date of supply at the time the supply is made: True or False?

88. The GMC number of a prescriber must be included on a private CD prescription: True or False?

89. Supervision on an instalment prescription is a legal requirement: True or False?

90. A pharmacist may request evidence of that person's identity if not already known to them when dispensing a schedule 2 or 3 CD prescription: True or False?

91. Midazolam and phenobarbital are not subject to safe custody: True or False?

92. For patient returned CDs an entry must be made in the CD register: True or False?

93. For CDs supplied, the name of the pharmacist supplying must be recorded in the CD register: True or False?

94. CD register entries must be made on the day of supply: True or False?

95. A CD running balance is not a legal requirement: True or False?

96. A statutory medical defence can be raised if driving is impaired and a specific drug is detected at higher levels than those permitted in the regulations, if there is evidence that the drug has been prescribed or bought and taken in accordance with the patient information leaflet: True or False?

97. The pharmacist's RPS number must be displayed on the RP notice: True or False?

98. The pharmacy record can be in writing, electronic or both: True or False?

99. The reason for any absence by the RP must be stated in the RP record: True or False?

100. If two pharmacists are working together, both can be RP at the same time: True or False?

101. GSL medicines can be sold in the absence of an RP but only if the RP is signed in: True or False?

Answers

1. GSL medicines can only be sold from a pharmacy: False

2. P medicines can be available for self-selection: False

3. A physiotherapist independent prescriber can prescribe schedule 2 CDs: True

4. It is unlawful to sell a product that contains more than 600 mg of pseudoephedrine: False

5. Advanced supply of EHC is allowed: True

6. Ulipristal acetate is only licensed for emergency contraception within 72 hours of unprotected sexual intercourse: False

7. The legal limit of paracetamol effervescent tablets that can be sold is 100: False

8. The maximum pack size for OTC dihydrocodeine is 16: False

9. The date of birth is a legal requirement on a prescription for a POM: False

10. The name of the prescriber is a legal requirement on a prescription: False

11. All prescriptions are valid for up to 6 months from the appropriate date: False

12. It is not a legal requirement for all prescriptions to be written in English: True

13. Private prescriptions for Schedule 4 and 5 CDs cannot be repeated: False

14. The first dispensing of a private POM prescription must be made within 6 months of the appropriate date, following which there is no legal time limit for the remaining repeats: True

15. NHS prescriptions can be repeated: False

16. Owings for co-codamol 30/500 tablets are valid for 28 days from the appropriate date: False

17. The name of the drug is a legal requirement for a POM: False

18. Private prescriptions for a POM must be retained for 2 years after dispensing: True

19. Private prescriptions for oral contraceptives are exempt from record keeping: True

20. The dose is a legal requirement when making a private prescription record in the POM register: False

21. Schedule 2, 3, 4 and 5 CD owings are valid for 28 days after the appropriate date: False

22. Faxed prescriptions are legal: False

23. Dentists are only legally allowed to prescribe medicines on the Dental Practitioners Formulary: False

24. Patients date of birth is a legal requirement on an EEA prescription: True

25. The Prescriber's email address is a legal requirement on an EEA prescription: True

26. The name of the drug is a legal requirement on an EEA prescription: True

27. EEA prescriptions are subject to prescription charges: False

28. Schedule 1, 2 and 3 CDs are not allowed on an EEA prescription: True

29. Emergency supply at the request of an EEA prescriber is allowed: True

30. Emergency supply at the request of an EEA patient for phenobarbital for epilepsy is allowed: False

31. It is a legal requirement for the name of the doctor to appear on a dispensing label: False

32. A patient specific direction is a written direction that allows the supply and/or administration of a specified medicine or medicines, by named authorised health professionals, to a well-defined group of patients requiring treatment for a specific condition: False

33. In an emergency, a pharmacist working in a registered pharmacy can supply POMs to a animal without a prescription: False

34. A podiatrist independent prescriber can request an emergency supply: True

35. In an emergency supply at the request of a prescriber, the prescriber must furnish a prescription within 48 hours: False

36. When making a POM register entry for an emergency supply at a request of a prescriber, two dates should be entered: False

37. Legislation prevents a pharmacist from making an emergency supply when the doctor's surgery is open: False

38. An emergency supply of phenobarbital in the UK can only be supplied for a maximum of 5 days: True

39. When making a POM register entry for emergency supply at the request of a prescriber, the dose is a legal requirement: False

40. All optometrists and podiatrists can authorise supplies of POMs by writing prescriptions: False

41. Any schoolteacher can sign a signed order to obtain salbutamol inhalers: False

42. The names of the students needing the salbutamol inhalers should be on the signed order: False

43. Appropriately headed paper must be used on a signed order for adrenaline auto-injectors for a school: False

44. Any pharmacist can supply nasal naloxone to a substance misuser without a prescription, PSD or PGD: False

45. All female patients wanting isotretinoin prescriptions must comply with PPP: False

46. Under the PPP, prescriptions for acitretin are valid for 7 days: True

47. All prescriptions for isotretinoin should only be prescribed for 30 days: False

48. Those planning pregnancies and taking valproate must schedule an appointment with their prescriber and stop taking valproate immediately: False

49. Lantus™ is an example of an original biologic medicine: True

50. A Pharmacist Independent Prescriber can prescribe unlicensed medicines subject to accepted good clinical practice: True

51. An optometrist independent prescriber can authorise an emergency supply for items that they can prescribe: True

52. A Vet can authorise an emergency supply for items that they can prescribe: False

53. Pharmacies can supply appropriate health professionals with a small number of POMs via

wholesale dealing as long as only a small profit is made: False

54. An independent nurse prescriber can be supplied with a small amount of medicines via wholesale dealing: False

55. POM-VPS are prescription-only medicines that can only be prescribed by a Vet and supplied by a Vet or pharmacist with a written prescription: False

56. A written prescription is needed to supply a NFA-VPS medicine: False

57. Vet prescriptions for Schedule 2, 3 and 4 drugs are valid for 28 days: True

58. The Veterinary Medicines Directorate advise that "as directed" is a legally acceptable dosage instruction on a vet prescription: False

59. Standardised forms are required for Vet schedule 2 and 3 CD prescriptions: False

60. Vet CD prescriptions should be sent to the relevant NHS agency: False

61. For all CDs, it is considered good practice for only 28 days' worth of treatment to be prescribed on a vet prescription: True

62. All vet prescriptions must include the Royal College of Veterinary Surgeons Registration number of the Vet: False

63. The cascade exemption within the Veterinary Medicines Regulations allows the supply of medicines that are not licensed for animals: True

64. It is lawful to sell human medicines for use in animals: False

65. The expiry date of a medicine supplied under the cascade must always be on the dispensing label: False

66. An entry must be made in the POM register for all POM-V and POM-VPS: False

67. Register entries for POM-V and POM-VPS can be kept electronically: True

68. Records and documents for POM-V and POM-VPS must be kept for two years: False

69. Animal adverse reactions and human adverse reactions to vet medicines should be reported to the MHRA: False

70. The Health Act 2006 introduced the concept of an accountable officer: True

71. There are two classes of Schedule 5 drugs: True

72. Sativex is a Schedule 4 Part II drug: False

73. Prescriptions for zopiclone are only valid for 28 days: True

74. The address of prescriber for a schedule 4 CD must be in the UK: False

75. NICE advise that organisations should consider retaining all CD invoices for six years for the purposes of HM Revenue and Customs: True

76. Pharmacists can, under one specific exemption, take possession of a schedule 1 CD: False

77. The name of supplier is a legal requirement for a CD requisition: False

78. The total quantity of a drug in words and figures is a legal requirement for a CD requisition: False

79. In an emergency, a doctor or dentist can be supplied with a Schedule 2 or 3 CD on the undertaking that a requisition will be supplied within the next 24 hours: True

80. When a requisition for a schedule 1, 2 or 3 CD is received, it is a legal requirement to mark the

requisition indelibly with the supplier's name and address: True

81. The person requesting the CD must send the original requisition to the relevant NHS agency: False

82. A registered midwife may use a midwife supply order to obtain diamorphine, morphine and oxycodone: False

83. The name of prescriber is a legal requirement on a prescription for a schedule 2 or 3 CD: False

84. The dose on a schedule 2 or 3 CD prescription does not need to be in words and figures: True

85. The name of drug is not a legal requirement on a schedule 2 or 3 CD prescription: True

86. It is a legal requirement for schedule 2, 3 or 4 CD prescriptions to not exceed a 30-day supply: False

87. When a schedule 2 or 3 CD is supplied, it is a requirement to mark the prescription with the date of supply at the time the supply is made: True

88. The GMC number of a prescriber must be included on a private CD prescription: False

89. Supervision on an instalment prescription is a legal requirement: False

90. A pharmacist may request evidence of that person's identity if not already known to them when dispensing a schedule 2 or 3 CD prescription: False

91. Midazolam and phenobarbital are not subject to safe custody: True

92. For patient returned CDs an entry must be made in the CD register: False

93. For CDs supplied, the name of the pharmacist supplying must be recorded in the CD register: False

94. CD register entries must be made on the day of supply: False

95. A CD running balance is not a legal requirement: True

96. A statutory medical defence can be raised if driving is impaired and a specific drug is detected at higher levels than those permitted in the regulations, if there is evidence that the drug has been prescribed or bought and taken in

accordance with the patient information leaflet: False

97. The pharmacist's RPS number must be displayed on the RP notice: False

98. The pharmacy record can be in writing, electronic or both: True

99. The reason for any absence by the RP in the RP record must be stated: False

100. If two pharmacists are working together, both can be RP at the same time: False

101. GSL medicines can be sold in the absence of an RP but only if the RP is signed in: True

Printed in Great Britain
by Amazon

71295595R00019